UNDERSTANDING YOUR EMOTIONS AND VALUES

A step-by-step guide to emotional management and self-values

Lawrence Armstrong

Table of contents

Chapter 1

Getting to meet yourself

The achievement of a point or purpose. Such a straightforward definition for a frequently mind-boggling and loaded thought. What is an accomplishment for you? Is it safe to say that you are taking a stab at an objective or accomplishment in light of outside proportions of progress or for the interior satisfaction of the most common way of gaining some new useful knowledge and exploring another test? These are difficult inquiries to respond to, however, they are fundamental for contemplating while thinking about how might affect you. As consultants, we urge understudies to look past the levels and outside criticism (while unquestionably significant) and inspect their inclinations, inclinations, values, and long-haul objectives as they think about a more extensive definition of individual achievement. What way will give you the most Pleasure, the most Fulfillment? How might you make a day-to-day existence that you would rather not escape from? Is the way that you are on, one that is in arrangement with your preferences? Will you be able to find a new line of work or get going on a satisfying profession? In this first section, we will provoke you to evaluate your ongoing way and consider your solutions to these inquiries determined to assist you with characterizing, or reclassifying how you will quantify your progress in school and throughout everyday life.

Recognizing you are why is an important step in identifying your path to success. The road to getting there may be different than you initially anticipated. It could veer very far from the version of success you were introduced to in your younger years.

It could also take you longer to get there than you hoped.

Chapter 2

Knowing your Values

Let's start with the definition of "personal value." Personal values are the things that are essential to us, the features and behaviors that inspire us and influence our actions.

For example, maybe you value honesty. You believe in being honest whenever possible, and you think it's necessary to communicate what you think. When you don't voice your thoughts, you probably feel disappointed in yourself.

Or maybe you appreciate compassion. You leap at the opportunity to assist other people, and you're generous in contributing your time and resources to important organizations or friends and family.

Those are only two instances of personal values out of countless. Everyone has their particular ideals, and they might be extremely diverse. Some individuals are competitive, while others appreciate collaboration. Some individuals cherish adventure, while others seek stability.

Values are important because you're likely to feel better if you're living according to your values and to feel worse if you don't. This applies both to day-to-day decisions and to broader life choices.

If you value adventure, for example, you'll undoubtedly feel limited if you let yourself be forced by parents or others into adopting "safe" choices like a solid office job and a settled home life. For you, a profession that includes travel, establishing your own company, or other possibilities for risk and excitement may be more suited.

On the other hand, if you prioritize security, the converse applies. What some people may consider a "dream" chance to travel the globe and be your boss may leave you feeling uncomfortable and desiring a more fixed lifestyle.

Everybody is different, and what makes one person happy may leave another feeling nervous or disconnected. Defining your unique values and then living by them may allow you to feel more satisfied and to make decisions that make you happy, even if they don't make sense to other people. You'll see how to go about achieving that in the next sections.

Chapter 3

Defining your Values

What makes you feel good? That's a wonderful place to start when figuring out what your values are. No, "ice cream" isn't a value. What we're talking about here are qualities or methods of acting in the world. As we saw before, someone who values honesty would feel good when they shared the truth.

Conversely, that same individual will feel horrible about themselves when they don't speak the truth. So unpleasant emotions may sometimes be an excellent signpost to your ideals. When have you felt disappointed in yourself or that you were a fraud? What behaviors lead up to that?

Here are some additional questions to get you started:

1. What's essential to you in life?

2. If you could have any job, without thinking about money or other practical restraints, what would you do?

3. When you're reading news headlines, what type of tale or conduct seems to inspire you?

4. What sort of tale or attitude gets you angry? What do you wish to change about the world or yourself?

5. What are you most proud of?

6. When were you the happiest?

Take a blank piece of paper and rapidly brainstorm some responses to these questions. Then use those responses as tools to figure out your ideals.

In certain circumstances, the values will be straightforward to figure out. If you typed "a loving relationship" in answer to the question about what's important to you, then "love" is an essential personal value for you.

If you wrote "being happy," then you value happiness.

Others may take a little more effort, however. For example, if you're motivated by tales of great entrepreneurs, maybe you value determination or accomplishment, or maybe it's riches and success. If you're motivated by activists striving to improve the world, maybe you value bravery or honesty, or maybe it's justice or peace. Try to evaluate what precisely it is about those tales or events that you connect to.

To assist you, here's a brief list of personal values:

- Achievement
- Adventure
- Courage
- Creativity
- Dependability
- Determination
- Friendship
- Health

- Honesty
- Independence
- Integrity
- Intelligence
- Justice
- Kindness
- Learning
- Love
- Peace
- Perfection
- Security
- Simplicity
- Sincerity
- Spontaneity
- Success
- Understanding
- Wealth

This is by no means a full collection of personal values. I'm sure you can think of many more. The objective isn't to choose things from a list, but to come up with your own based on your own experiences and personality.

 So, please use them as examples of personal ideals, but don't feel constrained by them. Let your creativity run wild!

When you've done brainstorming, you may have a half-dozen values, or you may have a vast list of dozens. If you're in the second camp, attempt to trim the list down to something manageable—perhaps 10 values that matter most to you. If you're suffering, try giving ratings to each one and then sorting the list in order.

Chapter 4

Keys to Emotion Management

Self-regulation is the capacity to experience your thoughts, feelings, and emotions and determine how you're going to behave in a manner that is beneficial for you and others.

Managing your emotions is a taught skill. it starts growing in infancy via your interaction with your major caregivers.

In reality, humans are born lacking the capacity to self-soothe. We depend on the neural systems of our caretakers to restore equilibrium, a process called co-regulation.

In reality, humans are born lacking the capacity to self-soothe. We depend on the neural systems of our caregivers to restore equilibrium.

When we are disturbed and dysregulated as newborns, laying on our caregiver's chest and synchronizing our breathing with theirs might help us calm down," she continues.

As we develop, the way our caregivers model emotional management, as well as the messages they offer us about our emotions, may have a great influence on how we perceive our emotions and whether we feel we can handle them," she says.

Teenagers and adults who did not encounter a supportive environment in early childhood may have a more difficult time with emotional control. If this sounds like you, don't despair. Several approaches may assist:

1. Take a deep breath

When you are overwhelmed with emotion, it's not feasible to think clearly and experience your emotions at the same time owing to the fight, flight, or freeze reaction going into high gear.

"Your pulse is likely speeding up, your blood supply to your belly and kidneys slows down, and adrenaline begins to rise.

When you're in this condition, it's difficult or impossible to understand what other people are saying, much alone being conscious of your thoughts and emotions. You're in survival mode for perceived danger.

Breath work may assist. Research suggests that deep breathing stimulates something called the parasympathetic nervous system (your "rest-and-digest" mode), which enables your body to relax and restore equilibrium.

Breathing Exercise:

You may find it beneficial to repeat this practice five or more times, or until relative calm is restored:

Inhale while counting to 4

Hold while counting to 4

Exhale while counting to 4

Hold while counting to 4

2. Sensory Grounding

When emotions are running strong, it may seem challenging to be present in your body or physical surroundings. If possible, attempt to tap into your five senses to remain grounded.

This may involve any variety of grounding tactics, such as spraying cold water on your face, chanting or humming, or adopting a technique called progressive muscular relaxation.

The 5-4-3-2-1 method:

5 things you can see

4 items you can touch

3 things you can hear

2 things you can smell

1 item you can taste.

Once you go through the workout, you've given yourself some diversion from your stressor and enabled your parasympathetic nervous system to kick in," she adds.

3. Mindfulness Activities

A daily meditation practice of 13 minutes for 8 weeks can enhance peoples' mood and emotional control, among other advantages.

Our brains contain neuroplasticity, which implies that they can alter and develop and adapt based on how we utilize them."

If meditation isn't your thing, you may also look at yoga, tai chi, gardening, or forest bathing as a resource.

4. Practice Embraciing your feelings

All too frequently, we describe feelings as "negative" or "bad." This might produce an extra layer of shame or guilt when you're already feeling emotionally heated.

Instead, you may find it beneficial to approach your sentiments from a position of inquiry rather than judgment. This is termed the "observer" attitude, or the condition of letting sensations ebb and flow, like the tide.

When you observe your emotions arising, it might be good to remark to yourself, "Isn't that interesting? I'm feeling fury. I allow it to be here, and I will get through this."

5. Enhance Your Self-Concept

If illogical beliefs are causing your emotional pain, you may find it beneficial to question them through cognitive reappraisal (changing the narrative).

Chapter 5

Enhance your Self-Concept

One of the most effective techniques for taking care of yourself is to create good and loving thoughts about understanding yourself. If we think well about understanding ourselves, we heal ourselves; and whatever prior scars that may be troubling us within become calmed.

Needless to say, this is one of the most crucial things we need to do to guarantee that we enjoy the trip of our life. If we have bad ideas about ourselves, we will take the anguish and inferiority complex inside ourselves into all the elements of our life and each one will be influenced negatively.

If we don't take the time to create a connection with ourselves and then verify the quality of ideas we think about regularly, this will not be achievable.

Undesirable thoughts about ourselves are the core reason behind a multitude of negative attitudes and actions. No plant with decaying roots is known to bloom nicely. People with weak self-esteem are unable to develop or keep nutritious connections in their life as they continually face internal unrest. The degree of the disruption will be in direct proportion to the amount of self-esteem.

Know when to express yourself

There's a time and place for everything, even deep emotions. Sobbing uncontrollably is a relatively frequent reaction to losing a loved one, for example. Screaming into your pillow, even hitting it, could help you express some rage and anxiety after being rejected.

Other instances, though, call for some moderation. No matter how furious you are, yelling at your supervisor over an unjust disciplinary action won't help.

Being attentive to your surroundings and the circumstance might help you understand when it's OK to let emotions out and when you might want to sit with them for the time.

Give yourself some space

Getting some space from overwhelming sensations might help you make sure you're responding to them in sensible ways, according to.

This distance could be physical, like leaving a distressing environment, for example. But you may also establish some mental space by diverting yourself.

Chapter 6

Knowing your Real Self

We have so much to say about the people around us. We spend vast amounts of energy and millions of thoughts throughout our lives thinking about the good and the poor attributes that other people possess. We don't leave anybody out, though, and even chat about total strangers (at times with great curiosity) (at times with great interest).

But there is someone we do tend to forget about, sometimes for large periods and sometimes for whole lives, and that person is concealed someplace deep inside our minds—ourselves. Knowing oneself will help you to realize your full potential to be happy, pleased, and fulfilled.

The only person we have the potential to manage and alter is ourselves and yet we spend so little time and energy on spending time thinking about ourselves.

- Nurture Yourself

If we don't provide time or attention to any element of our lives, it becomes ignored and suffers. Besides broad factors like economics, relationships, or profession (which are visibly influenced), this truth also holds for our bodies, our plants, our house, and even our pets. How can we, therefore, expect ourselves to grow without paying any conscious care or attention to it?

We drag ourselves from one worldly obligation to another and lose ourselves in the process, feeling depleted and sad. Just as a plant flowers when it receives enough care and attention, our 'Self' likewise blossoms when we take care of it like a small baby.

He lost his job and to his dismay was unable to crack any of the interviews he attended for. His self-esteem shattered and he had to move home with his parents to manage his life. He loathed associating with others after this experience because he believed that everyone looked down upon him and regarded him to be a loser.

His attitude grew so nasty that he could not even accept others for reasons of employment which further damaged his economic life. His sister saw this and counseled him on this as she knew his mind well. He understood his bad attitude and was determined to modify it after some soul-searching.

- Knowing Yourself

Form a connection with yourself to start with and investigate the type of thoughts you have for the most essential person in your life—YOU! Find the reason for the character of your thoughts and find techniques to shift those ideas around, if they happen to be negative.

High self-esteem creates the basis for a happy and positive existence and good ideas assist the establishment and upkeep of strong self-esteem.

Knowing oneself does not happen by merely spending time thinking about yourself. You need to ask yourself the correct questions to receive the all-important right answers.

You need to go about this healthily so that you don't wind up at the other extreme which is being obsessed with yourself. A few hints and the perfect words of guidance are all you need to become a self-aware human being.

Chapter 7

Ways to Becoming the Boss of Your Emotions:

1. Take a look at the influence of your emotions

Emotions make our lives interesting, distinctive, and vibrant,\s"Strong emotions might suggest that we embrace life completely, that we're not denying our natural reactions."

It's entirely natural to suffer some emotional overflow on occasion— when something fantastic occurs when something tragic happens when you feel like you've missed out.

So, how do you tell when there's a problem?

Emotions that routinely go out of control could lead to:

- connection or friendship conflict
- Difficulty connecting to others
- Trouble at work or school

- An inclination to use drugs to assist control your emotions
- physical or emotional outbursts

Find some time to take stock of precisely how your uncontrolled emotions are influencing your day-to-day existence. This will make it easy to identify problem areas measure your progress and track your success.

2. Aim for control, not Depression

You can't manage your emotions with a dial if it were that simple. But suppose, for a minute, you could regulate emotions this way.

You wouldn't want to keep them running at maximum all the time. You also wouldn't want to shut them off totally, though.

When you suppress or repress emotions, you're blocking yourself from experiencing and expressing them. This might happen intentionally through suppression or subconscious repression.

Either may lead to mental and physical health issues, including:

- Anxiety
- Depression
- Sleep difficulties
- Muscular strain and pain
- Difficulty managing stress
- Substance usage

When learning to exert control over emotions, be sure you aren't merely brushing them under the rug. Healthy emotional expression entails striking some balance between overpowering feelings and no emotions at all.

3. Identify what you're experiencing

Taking a minute to check in with yourself about your emotions will help you begin getting back control.

Say you've been seeing someone for a few months. You tried booking a date last week, but they indicated they didn't have time. Yesterday, you texted again, adding, "I'd want to meet you soon. Can you meet this week?"

They eventually react, more than a day later: "Can't. Busy."

You're suddenly terribly agitated. Without pausing to think, you fling your phone across the room, knock over your wastebasket, and kick your desk, stubbing your toe.

Interrupt yourself by asking:

What am I experiencing right now? disappointed, perplexed, furious What occurred to make me feel this way? They blew me off with no explanation.

Does the circumstance have an alternate explanation that would make sense? Maybe they're worried, unwell, or coping with something else they don't feel comfortable sharing. They could aim to explain more when they can.

What do I want to do about these feelings? (Scream, release my rage by tossing stuff, send back something unpleasant.

Is there a better method of dealing with them? Ask whether everything's OK. Ask when they're free next. Go for a stroll or run.

By examining different alternatives, you're reframing your thinking, which might help you adjust your original extreme response.

It might take some time before this reaction becomes a habit. With experience, going through these processes in your thoughts will become simpler (and more successful) (and more effective).

4. Talk to a therapist

If your emotions continue to seem overpowering, it may be time to seek professional assistance.

Long-term or chronic emotional dysregulation and mood fluctuations are connected to various mental health problems, including borderline personality disorder and bipolar disorder. Trouble managing emotions may also connect to trauma, familial troubles, or other underlying concerns, Botnick notes.

A therapist may give sympathetic, judgment-free assistance as you:

identify variables leading to dysregulated emotions

address severe mood swings learn how down-regulate intense feelings or up-regulate limited emotional expression practice challenging and reframing feelings that cause distress Mood swings and intense emotions can provoke negative or unwanted thoughts that eventually trigger feelings of hopelessness or despair.

This loop might ultimately lead to maladaptive coping mechanisms like self-harm or even thoughts of death. If you begin thinking about suicide or have cravings to self-harm, speak to a trusted loved one who can help you receive assistance right immediately